Slow Breakfast

Pressure Cooker Breakfast Recipes for Families

Nora J. Stewart

Sommario

Introduction

The Ninja Foodi multi-cooker is one of the home appliances that everyone must have in their kitchen. The gadget can replace 4 small tools: slow-moving stove, air fryer, pressure cooker and dehydrator.

This recipe book contains several of the recipes we have actually tried with the multi-cooker. The recipes range from morning meal, side meals, chicken, pork, soups, fish and shellfish, treats, and pasta. Additionally, we have actually compiled loads of vegetarian recipes you need to attempt. We created these dishes considering newbies and that's why the food preparation procedure is methodical. Besides, the dishes are tasty, enjoy reading.

Baked Omelet

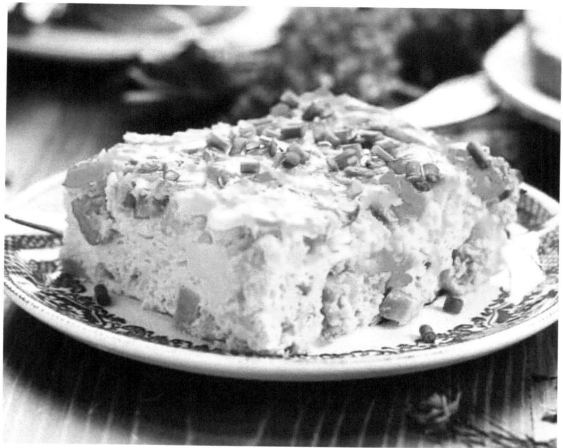

INGREDIENTS (6 Servings)

½ cup of milk
8 eggs
Kosher salt and pepper
1 cup of cheddar cheese, shredded
1 cup of cooked ham, diced
1/3 cup of green bell pepper, diced
1/3 cup of red bell pepper, diced
½ cup of fresh chives, diced

DIRECTIONS (PREP + COOK TIME: 45 MINUTES)

Close the crisping lid and preheat the unit on bake/ roast mode for 5 minutes having set the temperature to 315°F. Combine the milk with eggs, salt, and pepper in a bowl and add the remaining ingredients. Stir. Pour the mixture into a greased baking pan (8 inches) and place it on a rack. Place the rack in the preheated pot and close the crisping lid. Bake/roast the omelet on the same temperature settings for 35 minutes. Enjoy.

Bacon and Corn Bake
INGREDIENTS (6 Servings)

4 bacon slices, chopped
1 cup of cheddar cheese, grated
½ cup of heavy cream
 2 cups of corn
4 eggs, whisked
1 yellow onion, chopped
1 tablespoon of essential olive oil
1 teaspoon of thyme, chopped
2 teaspoons of garlic, grated
Salt and pepper

DIRECTIONS (PREP + COOK TIME: 45 MINUTES)
Set your Foodi to sauté mode, add oil, and allow it heat. Add the onions and cook for two minutes. Add the chopped bacon, corn, garlic, and thyme. Stir and cook for 5 minutes. Mix the remaining ingredients in the pot and close the crisping lid. Select the bake mode and set the cooking temperature to 320°F. Cook for twenty minutes and serve.

Almond Eggs
INGREDIENTS (4 Servings)

4 eggs, whisked
1 tablespoons of essential olive oil
1 red onion, chopped
3 oz. of almond milk
2 oz. of grated cheese
Splash of Worcestershire sauce

DIRECTIONS (PREP + COOK TIME: 20 MINUTES)

Select the sauté function on your Ninja Foodi. Add the oil and heat it. Add the chopped onions and stir. Cook for 5 minutes. Combine the remaining ingredients in a bowl and pour them over the sautéed onions. Stir the contents and close the crisping lid. Select the bake function, set temperatures to 375°F, and cook time to 10 minutes. Subdivide your almond eggs between plates and enjoy.

Banana Breakfast Mix
INGREDIENTS (6 Servings)

3 bananas (peeled and sliced)
1 egg, beaten
1 and ½ cups of coconut milk
2 glasses of rolled oats
½ cup of brown sugar
1 tablespoon of baking powder
1 teaspoon of vanilla extract
1 teaspoon of cinnamon powder
Cooking spray

DIRECTIONS (PREP + COOK TIME: 20 MINUTES)

Grease the Foodi pot lightly using the cooking spray. Add all the ingredients and close the pressure lid. Cook on high mode for 15 minutes. Allow the pressure to release naturally for 10 minutes. Quick release the remaining pressure and stir. Serve hot.

Cream Cheese and Bread

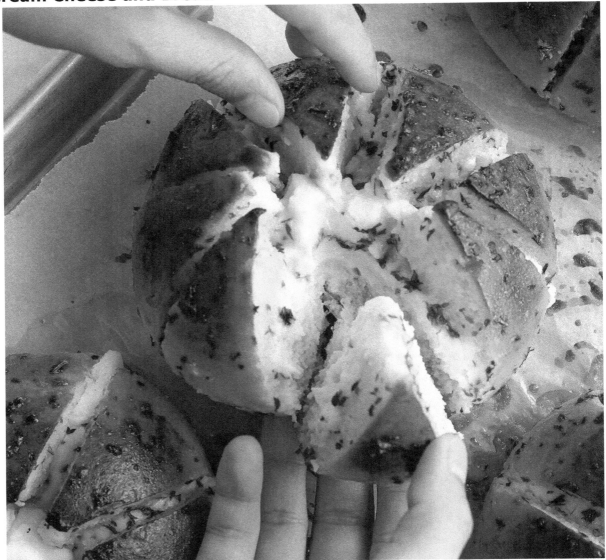

INGREDIENTS (6 Servings)

8 ounces of cream cheese
12 ounces of bread loaf, cubed
2 glasses of heavy cream
4 eggs
½ cup of brown sugar
1 teaspoon of cinnamon powder
1 teaspoon of vanilla flavoring
Cooking spray

DIRECTIONS (PREP + COOK TIME: 25 MINUTES)

Grease the baking pan with the cooking spray. Add all the ingredients and mix well. Place the reversible rack in the pot and put the rack on it. Close the crisping lid. Set the Foodi to air crisp mode and cook the ingredients over 325°F for 15 minutes. Subdivide your cheese delicacy amongst six plates.

Egg, Sausage, and Cheese Cake
INGREDIENTS (4 Servings)

8 eggs, beaten
8 oz. of breakfast sausage, chopped
3 slices of bacon, chopped
1 red bell pepper, chopped
1 green bell pepper, chopped
1 cup of green onion, chopped
1 cup of cheddar cheese, grated
1teaspoon of red chili flakes
½ cup of milk
4 bread slices,
½ inches cubed
2 cups of water
Salt and black pepper

DIRECTIONS (PREP + COOK TIME: 30 MINUTES)

Combine all the ingredients except the bread cubes and water in a bowl. Pour the egg mixture into a greased Bundt pan. Squeeze the bread cubes in the egg mixture using a spoon Pour water into the Ninja Foodi and insert the reversible rack. Place the pan on the rack and close the pressure lid. Ensure the release valve is set to seal position. Cook on high mode for 6 minutes and quick release the accumulated pressure. Slit the egg mixture using a knife and close the crisping lid. Cook on bake/roast mode for four minutes over the temperature of 380°F. Remove the egg mixture from the pan by inverting the pan over a platter. Slice the mixture and serve it alongside your preferred sauce.

Sweet Potato Eggs
INGREDIENTS (6 - 7 Servings)

2 tablespoons unsalted butter
1 yellow onion, diced
3 garlic cloves, minced
3 pounds sweet potatoes, diced
2 cups water 6 brown eggs
1 bunch scallions, sliced
1 red bell pepper, diced
1 green bell pepper, diced
2 teaspoons smoked paprika
Kosher salt
Ground black pepper

DIRECTIONS (Prep + Cook Time: 30-35 minutes)

Take Ninja Foodi multi-cooker, arrange it over a cooking platform, and open the top lid. In the pot, arrange a reversible rack and place the Crisping Basket over the rack. In the basket, add the potatoes. Seal the multi-cooker by locking it with the pressure lid; ensure to keep the pressure release valve locked/sealed. Select "PRESSURE" mode and select the "HI" pressure level. Then, set timer to 2 minutes and press "STOP/START"; it will start the cooking process by building up inside pressure. When the timer goes off, quickly release pressure by adjusting the pressure valve to the VENT. After pressure gets released, open the pressure lid. Remove the water and set aside the potatoes. In the pot, add the butter; Select the "SEAR/SAUTÉ" mode and select the "MD" pressure level. Press "STOP/START." Add the onions, garlic, bell peppers, and cook (while stirring) until they become softened for 4-5 minutes. Add the sweet potatoes, scallions, and paprika; stir-cook for 5 minutes. Season with salt and black pepper. Crack the eggs on top. Seal the multi-cooker by locking it with the crisping lid; ensure to keep the pressure release valve locked/sealed. Select the "AIR CRISP" mode and adjust the 325°F temperature level. Then, set timer to 10 minutes and press "STOP/START"; it will start the cooking process by building up inside pressure. When the timer goes off, quickly release pressure by adjusting the pressure valve to the VENT. After pressure gets released, open the Crisping Lid. Serve warm.

Onion And Mushroom Frittata
INGREDIENTS (4 Servings)

4 large eggs
¼ cup whole milk
Salt and pepper to taste
½ bell pepper, seeded and diced
½ onion, chopped
4 cremini mushrooms, sliced
½ cup shredded cheddar cheese

DIRECTIONS (Prep + Cook Time: 20 minutes)

Take a medium-sized bowl and whisk in eggs, milk and season with salt and pepper Add bell pepper, onion, mushroom, cheese and mix well Pre-heat Ninja Foodi by pressing the "BAKE" option and setting it to "400 Degrees F" and timer to 10 minutes Let it pre-heat until you hear a beep Pour Egg Mixture in the Ninja Foodi Bake Pan and spread well Transfer to Grill and lock lid, bake for 10 minutes until lightly golden Serve and enjoy!

Wholesome Mushroom Frittata
INGREDIENTS (4 Servings)

12 eggs; whisked
3 tablespoons olive oil
½ cup crème fraiche
1 cup cheddar cheese, shredded
8-ounce white mushrooms, sliced
2 leeks; chopped
1 cup water
2 tablespoons parsley; chopped
A pinch of salt and black pepper

DIRECTIONS (Prep + Cook Time: 25-30 minutes)

Take Ninja Foodi multi-cooker, arrange it over a cooking platform, and open the top lid. In the pot, add the oil; Select "SEAR/SAUTÉ" mode and select "MD: HI" pressure level. Press "STOP/START." After about 4-5 minutes, the oil will start simmering. Add the leeks, mushrooms, and cook (while stirring) until they become softened for 4-5 minutes. Add the mushrooms, stir-cook for 5 minutes. In a mixing bowl, whisk the eggs. Combine the crème Fraiche, parsley, salt, and pepper and whisk again. Add the mushroom mixture and combine again. Take a baking pan; grease it with some cooking spray, vegetable oil, or butter. Add the egg mixture in it and top with the cheese. Take Ninja Foodi multi-cooker, arrange it over a cooking platform, and open the top lid. In the pot, add water and place a reversible rack inside the pot. Place the pan over the rack. Seal the multi-cooker by locking it with the pressure lid; ensure to keep the pressure release valve locked/sealed. Select "PRESSURE" mode and select the "HI" pressure level. Then, set timer to 10 minutes and press "STOP/START"; it will start the cooking process by building up inside pressure. When the timer goes off, quickly release pressure by adjusting the pressure valve to the VENT. After pressure gets released, open the pressure lid. Serve warm.

Cheddar Tofu Breakfast
INGREDIENTS (4 Servings)

1 cup cheddar cheese, grated
2 medium onions, sliced
4 tablespoons full-fat butter
2 tofu blocks, cut into 1-inch pieces
Black pepper (ground) and salt to taste

DIRECTIONS (Prep + Cook Time: 18 minutes)

In a mixing bowl, add the tofu. Season with black pepper (ground) and salt. Combine the ingredients to mix well with each other. Take Ninja Foodi multi-cooker, arrange it over a cooking platform, and open the top lid. In the pot, add the butter; Select "SEAR/SAUTÉ" mode and select "MD: HI." pressure level. Press "STOP/START." After about 4-5 minutes, the butter will melt. Add the onions and cook (while stirring) until it becomes softened for 2-3 minutes. Add the seasoned tofu; stir-cook for 2 minutes more. Add the cheddar and gently stir the mixture. Seal the multi-cooker by locking it with the crisping lid; ensure to keep the pressure release valve locked/sealed. Select the "AIR CRISP" mode and adjust the 340°F temperature level. Then, set timer to 3 minutes and press "STOP/START"; it will start the cooking process by building up inside pressure. When the timer goes off, quick release pressure by adjusting the pressure valve to the VENT. After pressure gets released, open the crisping lid. Serve warm.

Buttermilk Omelet

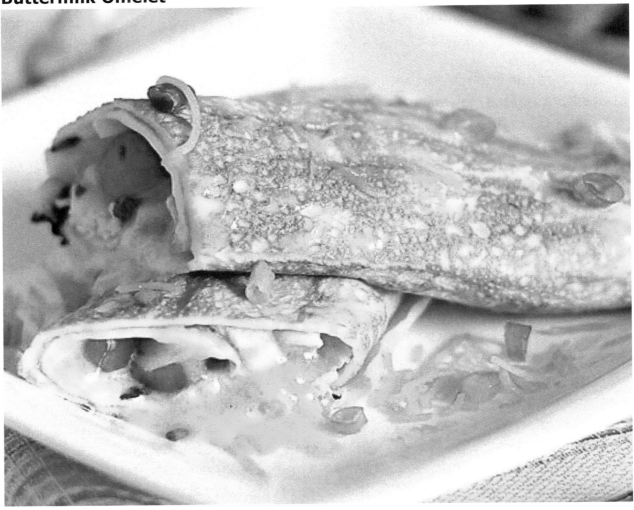

INGREDIENTS (4 Servings)

1 tablespoon basil; chopped
A pinch of black pepper (finely ground) and salt
4 eggs; whisked
1 cup buttermilk

DIRECTIONS (Prep + Cook Time: 15-20 minutes)

In a mixing bowl, mix all the ingredients and whisk well.   Take a baking pan; grease it with some cooking spray, vegetable oil, or butter. Add the mixture over it.   Take Ninja Foodi multi-cooker, arrange it over a cooking platform, and open the top lid.   In the pot, add water and place a reversible rack inside the pot. Place the pan over the rack. Seal the multi-cooker by locking it with the Crisping Lid; ensure to keep the pressure release valve locked/sealed. Select "BAKE/ROAST" mode and adjust the 400°F temperature level. Then, set timer to 10 minutes and press "STOP/START"; it will start the cooking process by building up inside pressure. When the timer goes off, quickly release pressure by adjusting the pressure valve to the VENT. After pressure gets released, open the Crisping Lid. Serve warm.

Blackberry Cornflakes
INGREDIENTS (4 Servings)

3 cups milk
2 eggs; whisked
4 tablespoons cream cheese, whipped
1 ½ cups corn flakes
¼ cup blackberries
1 tablespoon sugar
¼ teaspoon nutmeg, ground

DIRECTIONS (Prep + Cook Time: 15-20 minutes)

In a mixing bowl, mix all the ingredients and whisk well. Take a baking pan; grease it with some cooking spray, vegetable oil, or butter. Add the mixture over it. Take Ninja Foodi multi-cooker, arrange it over a cooking platform, and open the top lid. In the pot, add water and place a reversible rack inside the pot. Place the pan over the rack. Seal the multi-cooker by locking it with the Crisping Lid; ensure to keep the pressure release valve locked/sealed. Select "BAKE/ROAST" mode and adjust the 350°F temperature level. Then, set timer to 10 minutes and press "STOP/START"; it will start the cooking process by building up inside pressure. When the timer goes off, quickly release pressure by adjusting the pressure valve to the VENT. After pressure gets released, open the Crisping Lid. Serve warm.

Tofu with Mixed Veggies
INGREDIENTS (4 Servings)

2 tablespoons of essential olive oil
1 package (16-oz) of extra-firm tofu (drained and pressed)
½ onion, sliced
½ zucchini, chopped
 ½ green bell pepper, chopped
1 cup of broccoli, chopped
1 can (14.5-oz) of diced tomatoes
½ teaspoon of dried rosemary
¼ cup of vegetable broth
1 teaspoon of dried thyme
1 pinch of dried basil
½ teaspoon of oregano
Ground black pepper
¼ cup of nutritional yeast

DIRECTIONS (PREP + COOK TIME: 32 MINUTES)
Wrap tofu in paper towels and press it for 5 minutes. Cut it into bite-size pieces. Sauté the tofu pieces until they turn light brown. Add garlic, onions and bell pepper. Let it cook for 3 minutes. Add the zucchini, tomatoes, broccoli, and herbs. Close the pressure lid and cook 4 minutes. Quick release the accumulated pressure and serve. Sprinkle each plate with black pepper and yeast.

Deli Salmon Veggies Cakes
INGREDIENTS (4 Servings)

25-oz of packed salmon flakes (steamed)
1cup of breadcrumbs
1 red onion, finely diced
1 red pepper (seeded and diced)
4 tablespoons of butter, divided
4 tablespoons of mayonnaise
2 teaspoons of Worcestershire sauce
¼ cup of parsley, chopped
1 teaspoon of garlic powder
2 teaspoons of olive oil
Salt and black pepper
3 eggs, beaten
3 large potatoes cut into chips

DIRECTIONS (PREP + COOK TIME: 35 MINUTES)
Preheat the Foodi by setting it to sauté mode. Add the oil and butter. Sauté the contents until the butter melt. Add the onions and red pepper. Let it cook for 6 minutes and turn off the sauté mode. Combine the salmon flakes with breadcrumbs, garlic powder, Worcestershire sauce, mayonnaise, parsley, salt, black pepper, sautéed red bell pepper, and onions in a bowl. Mix well using a spoon to breakdown the salmon. Form 4 patties from the mixture and add the remaining butter. Fry for 5 minutes to melt the butter while flipping. Close the crisping lid and bake/roast for 4 minutes at 320°F. Serve your cake with salad. You can also spray it with herb vinaigrette for additional flavor.

Breakfast Roll Casserole
INGREDIENTS (4 Servings)

12 eggs
1 cup of milk A crescent roll, halved
½ pound of pork sausage, cooked
Salt and Pepper

DIRECTIONS (PREP + COOK TIME: 25 MINUTES)
Mole the halved crescent rolls into balls and set aside. Cook the sausage and drain it using towels. Put all the ingredients into the Ninja Foodi except the reserved rolls. Now, add the crescent roll balls and close the pressure lid. Set the release valve to seal position and cook on high mode for 15 minutes. Release the in-built pressure naturally and open the pressure lid. Serve hot.

Turmeric Cauliflower
INGREDIENTS (4 Servings)

2 cups of cauliflower florets
1 cup of veggie stock
A handful of cilantro, chopped.
2 garlic cloves, minced.
2 tablespoons of essential olive oil
2 tablespoons of turmeric powder
Salt and black pepper

DIRECTIONS (PREP + COOK TIME: 30 MINUTES)

Set the Foodi to Sauté mode and add oil. Heat it and add the garlic. Cook for a minute. Add all the ingredients to the pot (except the cilantro) and toss. Set your multi-cooker to baking mode and cook at 380 °F for 20 minutes. Add the cilantro and toss. Subdivide your turmeric cauliflower amongst plates as a side dish.

Zucchini Spaghetti
INGREDIENTS (4 Servings)

3 zucchinis cut with a spiralizer
1 cup of sweet peas
1 cup of cherry tomatoes, halved
6 basil leaves, torn
1 tablespoon of extra virgin olive oil
A pinch of salt and black pepper
spaghetti
For the pesto:
1/3 cup of pine nuts
¼ cup of parmesan, grated
½ cup of extra virgin olive oil
3 cups of basil leaves
2 garlic cloves
A pinch of salt and black pepper

DIRECTIONS (PREP + COOK TIME: 10 MINUTES)

Mix ½ tablespoon of oil with 3 cups basil, garlic, pine nuts, parmesan, salt, and pepper in a blender. Pulse well. Set the Foodi to sauté mode and add the remaining oil. Heat it up. Add the zucchini, spaghetti, peas, tomatoes, and the pesto. Toss and close the pressure lid. Cook on high mode for 5 minutes. Release the in-built pressure naturally for four minutes and quick release the rest. Open the lid and add the torn basil leaves. Toss and subdivide your zucchini spaghetti between plates as a side dish.

Brussels sprouts

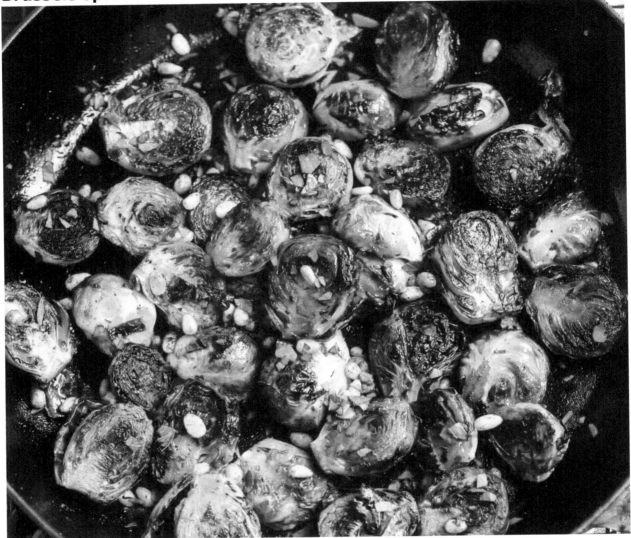

INGREDIENTS (4 Servings)

1 lb of Brussels sprouts (trimmed and halved)
2 tablespoons of garlic, minced
6 teaspoons of extra virgin olive oil
Salt and black pepper

DIRECTIONS (PREP + COOK TIME: 22 MINUTES)

Put all the ingredients into your Foodi's air crisp basket. Stir. Insert the basket into the multi-cooker and set it to air crisp mode. Cook the sprouts at 400 °F for 12 minutes. Subdivide your Brussels sprouts between plates as a side dish.

Baby Carrots
INGREDIENTS (4 Servings)

1 lb of baby carrots, trimmed
2 tablespoons of lime juice
2 teaspoons of essential olive oil
1 teaspoons of herbs de Provence

DIRECTIONS (PREP + COOK TIME: 25 MINUTES)
Put all the ingredients into a bowl and toss. Transfer them into a crisping basket and fix it in the Foodi. Add the trimmed carrots and close the crisping lid. Air-fry the mixture at 350 °F for 15 minutes. Subdivide your carrot side dish between plates.

Herbed Sweet Potatoes
INGREDIENTS (6 Servings)

3 lb of sweet potatoes, wedged
½ cup of parmesan, grated
2 garlic cloves
2 tablespoons of butter, melted
½ teaspoon of parsley, dried
¼ teaspoon of sage, dried
½ tablespoon of rosemary, dried
Salt and black pepper

DIRECTIONS (PREP + COOK TIME: 25 MINUTES)
Combine all the ingredients in the Foodi's baking dish. Toss. Insert the reversible rack in the pot and place the baking dish on it. Set the multi-cooker to baking mode and cook at 360 °F for 20 minute. Divide the sweet potatoes side dish between plates and enjoy.

Buttery Broccoli
INGREDIENTS (4 Servings)

1 broccoli head, florets separated
½ cup of chicken stock
½ cup of parmesan, grated
2 garlic cloves, minced
1 yellow onion, chopped
2 tablespoons of parsley, chopped
3 tablespoons of butter
Salt and black pepper

DIRECTIONS (PREP + COOK TIME: 35 MINUTES)
Set the Foodi to Sauté mode and add the butter. Melt it. Add onions and the garlic. Stir and cook for 5 minutes   Add the remaining ingredients (except the parsley and the parmesan) and toss. Set your Foodi to baking mode and cook at 360 °F for 20 minutes. Sprinkle it with cheese and parmesan. Toss and subdivide the buttery side dish between plates.

Buttery Mushrooms
INGREDIENTS (4 Servings)

1 lb of button mushrooms, halved
3 tablespoons of butter, melted
2 tablespoons of parmesan, grated
1 teaspoon of Italian seasoning
A pinch of salt and black pepper

DIRECTIONS (PREP + COOK TIME: 20 MINUTES) Set the Foodi to Sauté mode and add butter. Heat it up to melt. Add the mushrooms followed by the remaining ingredients and toss. Close the pressure cooking lid and cook on high mode for 10 minutes. Release the pressure naturally for 10 minutes. Subdivide the buttery mushroom between serving plates as a side dish.

INGREDIENTS (4 Servings)

1 cup of veggie stock
2 tablespoons of butter, melted
2 tablespoons of sour cream
1 butternut squash (peeled and cubed)
Salt and black pepper

DIRECTIONS (PREP + COOK TIME: 30 MINUTES) Mix the squash with the stock, salt, and pepper in your Foodi. Toss and close the pressure lid. Cook on high mode for twenty minutes Release the stress naturally for 10 minutes. Mash the squash well and add butter followed by the sour cream. Whisk well and subdivide the mash between four serving plates a side dish.

Red Cabbage
INGREDIENTS (2 Servings)

1 red cabbage head, shredded
1 cup of sour cream
1 red onion, chopped
4 bacons (sliced and chopped)
Salt and black pepper

DIRECTIONS (PREP + COOK TIME: 30 MINUTES) Set the Foodi to sauté mode and add the bacon. Stir and brown it for four minutes. Add onions, cabbages, salt, and pepper to the bacon. Stir and cook for four minutes. Add the sour cream and toss well. Close the pressure lid and cook on high mode for 12 minutes. Release the pressure naturally for ten minutes. Subdivide your red cabbage between the serving plates as a side dish.

Mexican Beans

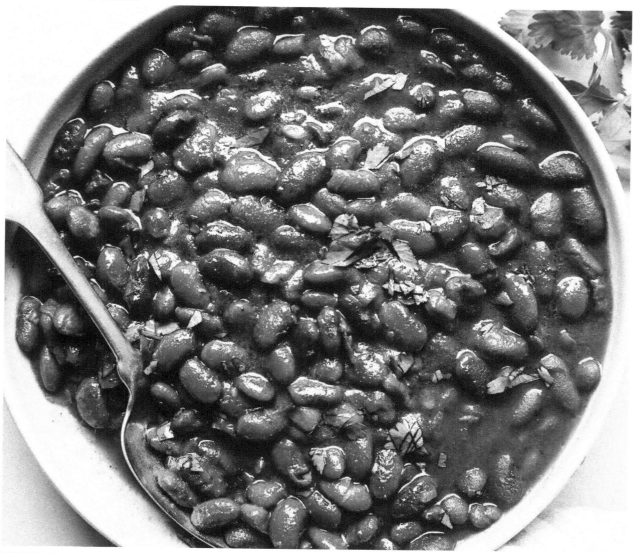

INGREDIENTS (4 Servings)

A cup of canned garbanzo beans, drained
1 cup of canned cranberry beans, drained
A cup of chicken stock
1 bunch of parsley, chopped
1 small red onion, chopped
1 garlic herb, minced
2 celery stalks, chopped
5 tablespoons of apple cider vinegar
4 tablespoons of organic olive oil

Salt and black pepper

DIRECTIONS (PREP + COOK TIME: 30 MINUTES)

Set the Foodi to sauté mode and add the oil. Heat it up and add onions and the minced garlic. Stir and sauté the seasonings for 5 minutes. Add the remaining ingredients and toss. Close the pressure lid and cook on high mode for 15 minutes. Natural-release the accumulated moisture and open the lid. Subdivide your Mexican beans between serving plates as a side dish.

Oregano Potatoes
INGREDIENTS (2 Servings)

4 gold potatoes (cut into wedges)
4 garlic cloves, minced
½ cup of water
2 tablespoons of essential olive oil
1 tablespoon of oregano, chopped
Juice extracted from a lemon
 A pinch of salt and black pepper

DIRECTIONS (PREP + COOK TIME: 35 MINUTES)
Pour water into the Foodi and insert a basket into it. Put potatoes in the basket and close the pressure lid. Cook it on low mode for four minutes. Release the pressure naturally for 10 minutes and drain the potatoes. Transfer them to a large bowl and set aside. Clean the Ninja pot and set it to sauté mode. Add oil and heat. Add the potatoes followed by the remaining ingredients and toss. Set the Foodi to roast mode and cook at 400 °F for twenty minutes. Subdivide your oregano potatoes between serving plates and enjoy.

Baked Mushrooms
INGREDIENTS (4 Servings)

1 lb of white mushrooms, halved
1 tablespoon of oregano, chopped
2 tablespoons of mozzarella cheese, grated
2 tablespoons of organic olive oil
1 tablespoon of parsley, chopped
1 tablespoon of rosemary, chopped
Salt and black pepper

DIRECTIONS (PREP + COOK TIME: 25 MINUTES)

Set the Foodi to sauté mode and add the oil. Heat it up and mix all the ingredients (except cheese.) Spread the grated cheese over the mixture and set the Foodi to baking mode. Cook the mushrooms mixture over 380 °F for 15 minutes. Subdivide your mushroom side dish between plates as a side dish

Paprika Beets
INGREDIENTS (4 Servings)

2 lbs of small beets (trimmed and halved)
1 tablespoon of olive oil
 4 tablespoons of sweet paprika

DIRECTIONS (PREP + COOK TIME: 45 MINUTES)
Mix all the ingredients in a bowl. Put the beets in the crisping basket and insert it into the Foodi. Set the multi-cooker to air crisp mode and cook the beets over 380 °F for 35 minutes. Subdivide your beets between serving plates as a side dish.

Broccoli Mash
INGREDIENTS (4 Servings)

1 broccoli head (florets separated and steamed)
½ cup of veggie stock
½ teaspoon of turmeric powder
1 tablespoon of olive oil
A tablespoon of chives, chopped
1 tablespoon of butter, melted
Salt and black pepper

DIRECTIONS (PREP + COOK TIME: 21 MINUTES)
Set the Foodi to sauté mode and add the oil. Heat it up and add the broccoli florets. Cook them for 4 minutes. Add the remaining ingredients (except butter and chives) and close the pressure lid. Cook everything on high mode for 12 minutes. Release the pressure naturally for ten minutes. Mash the cooked broccoli and add butter and chives. Stir your broccoli mash and subdivide it between plates.

Cumin Green Beans
INGREDIENTS (6 Servings)

1 lb of green beans, trimmed
2 garlic cloves, minced
1 tablespoon of olive oil
½ teaspoon of cumin seeds
Salt and black pepper

DIRECTIONS (PREP + COOK TIME: 20 MINUTES)

Combine all the ingredients in a bowl and toss well. Transfer the green beans mixture to a crisping basket and insert it in the Foodi. Set the appliance to air crisp mode and cook the mixture over 370 °F for 15 minutes, Subdivide the side dish between plates and enjoy.

Carrot Fries

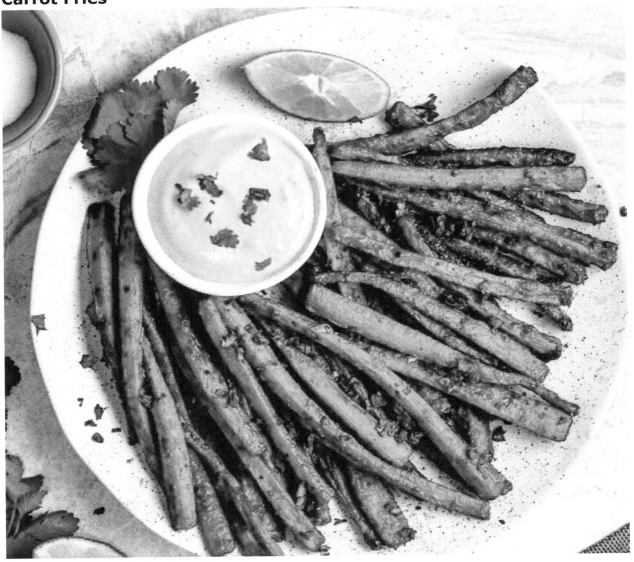

INGREDIENTS (4 Servings)

4 mixed carrots cut into sticks
2 garlic cloves, minced
2 tablespoons of rosemary, chopped
2 tablespoons of olive oil
Salt and black pepper

DIRECTIONS (PREP + COOK TIME: 25 MINUTES)

Mix all the ingredients in a bowl. Transfer the carrot mixture into an air crisp basket and fix it in the Foodi. Set the multi-cooker to air crisp mode and cook the fries over 380 °F for fifteen minutes. Subdivide your carrot fries between plates and serve as a side dish

Peanut Butter And Banana Chips
INGREDIENTS (4 Servings)

2 bananas, sliced into ¼ inch rounds
2 tablespoons creamy peanut butter

DIRECTIONS (Prep + Cook Time: 8 hours 10 minutes)
Take a medium-sized bowl and add banana slices with peanut butter, toss well until coated If the butter is too thick, add 1-2 tablespoons water Place banana slices flat on your Crisper Basket and arrange them in a single layer Transfer basket to your Grill Grate Pre-heat Ninja Foodi by pressing the "DEHYDRATE" option and setting it to "135 Degrees F" and timer to 15 minutes Let it pre-heat until you hear a beep Let them dehydrate until the default timer runs out Once done, store them In Air Tight container and serve when needed Enjoy!

Blistered Green Beans
INGREDIENTS (4 Servings)

1-pound green beans, trimmed
2 tablespoons vegetable oil
1 lemon, juiced
Pinch of red pepper flakes
Flaky sea salt as needed
Fresh ground black pepper as needed

DIRECTIONS (Prep + Cook Time: 15 minutes)
Take a medium-sized bowl and add green beans Pre-heat Ninja Foodi by pressing the "GRILL" option and setting it to "MAX" and timer to 10 minutes Let it pre-heat until you hear a beep Once preheated, transfer green beans to Grill Grate Lock lid and let them grill for 8-10 minutes, making sure to toss them from time to time until all sides are blustered well Squeeze lemon juice over green beans and top with red pepper flakes, season with salt and pepper.

Jalapeno Tomato Eggs
INGREDIENTS (4 Servings)

½ medium red or green bell pepper, seeded and chopped
1 medium jalapeño pepper, seeded and minced
3 tablespoons olive oil
1 small onion, chopped
2 garlic cloves, chopped
1 teaspoon kosher salt
½ teaspoon ground cumin
½ teaspoon smoked paprika
½ teaspoon red pepper flakes
¼ teaspoon ground black pepper
2 (14.5 ounce) cans diced tomatoes with their juice
4 large eggs
⅓ cup crumbled feta cheese (optional)
2 tablespoons chopped parsley

DIRECTIONS (Prep + Cook Time: 15-20 minutes)

Take Ninja Foodi multi-cooker, arrange it over a cooking platform, and open the top lid. In the pot, add the oil; Select "SEAR/SAUTÉ" mode and select "MD: HI" pressure level. Press "STOP/START." After about 4-5 minutes, the oil will start simmering. Add the onions, salt, bell pepper, jalapeño, garlic, and cook (while stirring) until they become softened and translucent for 2-3 minutes. Add the tomatoes, cumin, paprika, red pepper flakes, and black pepper. Stir gently. Seal the multi-cooker by locking it with the pressure lid; ensure to keep the pressure release valve locked/sealed. Select "PRESSURE" mode and select the "HI" pressure level. Then, set timer to 4 minutes and press "STOP/START"; it will start the cooking process by building up inside pressure. When the timer goes off, quick release pressure by adjusting the pressure valve to VENT. After pressure gets released, open the pressure lid. Gently crack the eggs over. Seal the multi-cooker by locking it with the pressure lid; ensure to keep the pressure release valve locked/sealed. Select "STEAM" mode. Then, set timer to 3 minutes. Serve with the cheese and parsley on top.

Ham Spinach Breakfast
INGREDIENTS (6 Servings)

4 cups ham, sliced
4 tablespoons butter, melted
3 pounds baby spinach
½ cup full-fat cream
Salt and black pepper to taste

DIRECTIONS (Prep + Cook Time: 20 minutes)

Take Ninja Foodi multi-cooker, arrange it over a cooking platform, and open the top lid. In the pot, add the butter; Select "SEAR/SAUTÉ" mode and select "MD: HI." pressure level. Press "STOP/START." After about 4-5 minutes, the butter will melt. Add the spinach and cook (while stirring) until it becomes softened for 2-3 minutes. Top with the cream, ham slices, black pepper (ground), and salt. Seal the multi-cooker by locking it with the crisping lid; ensure to keep the pressure release valve locked/sealed. Select "BAKE/ROAST" mode and adjust the 360°F temperature level. Then, set timer to 8 minutes and press "STOP/START"; it will start cooking process by building up inside pressure. When the timer goes off, quick release pressure by adjusting the pressure valve to the VENT. After pressure gets released, open the crisping lid. Serve warm.

Zucchini Egg Omelet
INGREDIENTS (2 Servings)

4 eggs ¼ teaspoon basil, chopped
¼ teaspoon red pepper flakes, crushed
1 teaspoon full-fat butter
1 zucchini, julienned
Salt and ground black pepper to taste preference

DIRECTIONS (Prep + Cook Time: 20-25 minutes)

Take Ninja Foodi multi-cooker, arrange it over a cooking platform, and open the top lid. In the pot, add the butter; Select "SEAR/SAUTÉ" mode and select "MD: HI." pressure level. Press "STOP/START." After about 4-5 minutes, the butter will melt. Add the zucchini and cook (while stirring) until it becomes softened for 4-5 minutes. In a mixing bowl, beat the eggs. Add the basil, red pepper flakes, salt, and black pepper; combine the ingredients to mix well with each other. Add the egg mixture over zucchini and stir the mixture. Seal the multi-cooker by locking it with the crisping lid; ensure to keep the pressure release valve locked/sealed. Select the "AIR CRISP" mode and adjust the 355°F temperature level. Then, set timer to 10 minutes and press "STOP/START"; it will start the cooking process by building up inside pressure. When the timer goes off, quick release pressure by adjusting the pressure valve to the VENT. After pressure gets released, open the crisping lid. Slice into wedges and serve warm.

Classic Butter Eggs

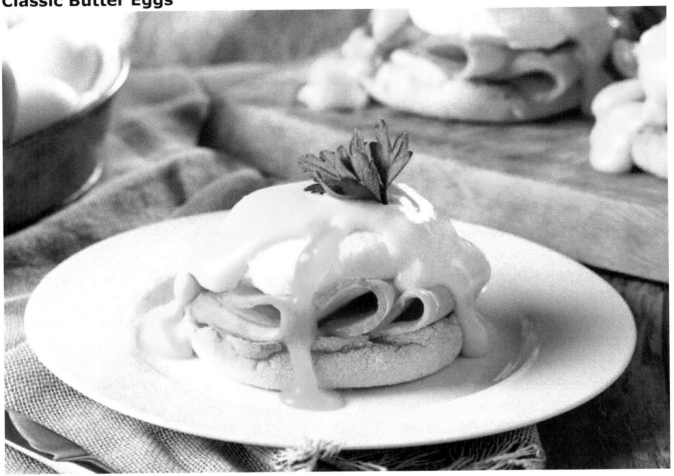

INGREDIENTS (2 Servings)

1 teaspoon butter, melted
¾ teaspoon salt
4 eggs
¼ teaspoon ground black pepper

DIRECTIONS (Prep + Cook Time: 15-20 minutes)

Take a baking pan; grease it with some butter. Beat the eggs and add in the pan. Add the melted butter on top. Season with the ground black pepper and salt. Seal the multi-cooker by locking it with the crisping lid; ensure to keep the pressure release valve locked/sealed. Select the "AIR CRISP" mode and adjust the 350°F temperature level. Then, set timer to 10 minutes and press "STOP/START"; it will start the cooking process by building up inside

50

pressure.   When the timer goes off, quick release pressure by adjusting the pressure valve to the VENT.   After pressure gets released, open the crisping lid. Optionally serve with steamed broccoli, spinach, or asparagus on the side.

Breakfast Bundt Cake
INGREDIENTS (7-8 Servings)

¼ teaspoon cinnamon
¼ teaspoon sea salt
2 cups all-purpose flour
1 teaspoon baking soda
1 stick unsalted butter
2 eggs, beaten
1 teaspoon vanilla extract
3 ripe bananas, mashed
½ cup dark brown sugar
¼ cup granulated sugar
1 cup chocolate chips, semisweet

DIRECTIONS (Prep + Cook Time: 45-50 minutes)
In a mixing bowl, combine the flour, baking soda, cinnamon, and salt. In another bowl, whisk the butter, brown sugar, and granulated sugar. Add the eggs, vanilla, and bananas; stir again. Combine both the mixture and mix in the chocolate chips. Take a 7-inch Bundt pan; grease it with some cooking spray, vegetable oil, or butter. Pour the batter into the pan. Take Ninja Foodi multi-cooker, arrange it over a cooking platform, and open the top lid. In the pot, add water and place a reversible rack inside the pot. Place the pan over the rack. Seal the multi-cooker by locking it with the Crisping Lid; ensure to keep the pressure release valve locked/sealed. Select "BAKE/ROAST" mode and adjust the 325°F temperature level. Then, set timer to 30 minutes and press "STOP/START"; it will start the cooking process by building up inside pressure. When the timer goes off, quickly release pressure by adjusting the pressure valve to the VENT. After pressure gets released, open the Crisping Lid. If needed, bake for 10 more minutes. The toothpick inserted should come out clean and dry. Serve warm.

Pumpkin Porridge
INGREDIENTS (8 Servings)

1 cup unsweetened almond milk, divided
2 pounds pumpkin, peeled and cubed into ½-inch size
6-8 drops liquid stevia
½ teaspoon ground allspice
1 tablespoon ground cinnamon
1 teaspoon ground nutmeg
¼ teaspoon ground cloves
½ cup walnuts, chopped

DIRECTIONS (Prep + Cook Time: 5 hours 15 minutes)
In the pot of Ninja Foodie, place ½ cup of almond milk and remaining ingredients and stir to combine. Close the Ninja Foodi with a crisping lid and select "Slow Cooker." Set on "Low" for 4-5 hours. Press "Start/Stop" to begin cooking. Open the lid and stir in the remaining almond milk. With a potato masher, mash the mixture completely. Divide the porridge into serving bowls evenly. Serve warm with the topping of walnuts.

Dried Fruit Oatmeal
INGREDIENTS (8 Servings)

2 cups steel-cut oats
1/3 cup dried apricots, chopped
1/3 cup raisins
1/3 cup dried cherries
1 teaspoon ground cinnamon
4 cups milk
4 cups water
¼ teaspoon liquid stevia

DIRECTIONS (Prep + Cook Time: 8 hours 10 minutes) In the pot of Ninja Foodie, place all ingredients and stir to combine. Close the Ninja Foodi with a crisping lid and select "Slow Cooker." Set on "Low" for 6-8 hours. Press "Start/Stop" to begin cooking. Open the lid and serve warm.

Eggs in Avocado Cups
INGREDIENTS (2 Servings)

1 avocado, halved and pitted
Salt and ground black pepper, as required
2 eggs
1 tablespoon Parmesan cheese, shredded
1 teaspoon fresh chives, minced

DIRECTIONS (Prep + Cook Time: 17 minutes)
Arrange a greased square piece of foil in "Cook & Crisp Basket." Arrange the "Cook & Crisp Basket" in the pot of Ninja Foodi. Close the Ninja Foodi with a crisping lid and select "Bake/Roast." Set the temperature to 390 degrees F for 5 minutes. Press "Start/Stop" to begin preheating. Carefully scoop out about 2 teaspoons of flesh from each avocado half. Crack 1 egg in each avocado half and sprinkle with salt, black pepper, and cheese. After preheating, open the lid. Place the avocado halves into the "Cook & Crisp Basket." Close the Ninja Foodi with a crisping lid and Select "Bake/Roast." Set the temperature to 390 degrees F for 12 minutes. Press "Start/Stop" to begin cooking. Open the lid and transfer the avocado halves onto serving plates. Top with Parmesan and chives and serve.

Chicken Omelet
INGREDIENTS (2 Servings)

1 teaspoon butter
1 small yellow onion, chopped
½ jalapeño pepper, seeded and chopped
3 eggs
Salt and ground black pepper, as required
¼ cup cooked chicken, shredded

DIRECTIONS (Prep + Cook Time: 26 minutes)

Select the "Sauté/Sear" setting of Ninja Foodi and place the butter into the pot. Press "Start/Stop" to begin cooking and heat for about 2-3 minutes. Add the onion and cook for about 4-5 minutes. Add the jalapeño pepper and cook for about 1 minute. Meanwhile, in a bowl, add the eggs, salt, and black pepper and beat well. Press "Start/Stop" to stop cooking and stir in the chicken. Top with the egg mixture evenly. Close the Ninja Foodi with a crisping lid and select "Air Crisp." Set the temperature to 355 degrees F for 5 minutes. Press "Start/Stop" to begin cooking. Open the lid and transfer the omelet onto a plate. Cut into equal-sized wedges and serve hot.

Sausage & Bell Pepper Frittata

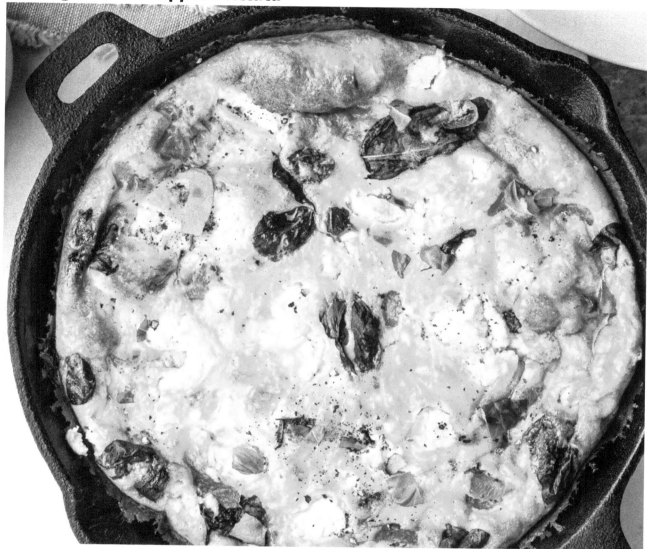

INGREDIENTS (2 Servings)

1 tablespoon olive oil
1 chorizo sausage, sliced
1½ cups bell peppers, seeded and chopped
4 large eggs
Salt and ground black pepper, as required
2 tablespoons feta cheese, crumbled
1 tablespoon fresh parsley, chopped

DIRECTIONS (Prep + Cook Time: 33 minutes) Select the "Sauté/Sear" setting of Ninja Foodi and place the butter into the pot. Press "Start/Stop" to begin cooking and heat for about 2-3 minutes. Add the sausage and bell peppers and cook for 6-8 minutes or until golden brown. Meanwhile, in a small bowl, add the eggs, salt, and black pepper and beat well. Press "Start/Stop" to stop cooking and place the eggs over the sausage mixture, followed by the cheese and parsley. Close the Ninja Foodi with a crisping lid and select "Air Crisp." Set the temperature to 355 degrees F for 10 minutes. Press "Start/Stop" to begin cooking. Open the lid and transfer the frittata onto a platter. Cut into equal-sized wedges and serve hot.

Eggs with Tomatoes
INGREDIENTS (6 Servings)

1 tablespoon olive oil
1 medium yellow onion, chopped
2 garlic cloves, minced
1 jalapeño pepper, seeded and chopped finely
2 teaspoons smoked paprika
1 teaspoon ground cumin
Salt, as required
1 (26-ounce) can diced tomatoes
6 eggs
¼ cup feta cheese, crumbled

DIRECTIONS (Prep + Cook Time: 8 hours 40 minutes) Select the "Sauté/Sear" setting of Ninja Foodi and place the butter into the pot. Press "Start/Stop" to begin cooking and heat for about 2-3 minutes. Add the onion and cook for about 3-4 minutes. Add the garlic, jalapeño, paprika, cumin, and salt and cook for about 1 minute. Press "Start/Stop" to stop cooking. Close the Ninja Foodi with a crisping lid and select "Slow Cooker." Set on "Low" for 8 hours. Press "Start/Stop" to begin cooking. Open the lid and with the back of a spoon, make 6 wells in the tomato mixture. Carefully crack 1 egg in each well. Close the Ninja Foodi with a crisping lid and select "Slow Cooker."Set on "High" for 20 minutes. Press "Start/Stop" to begin cooking. Open the lid and serve hot with the topping of cheese.

Hash Brown Casserole
INGREDIENTS (1 Servings)

3 tablespoons of organic olive oil
48 oz. of frozen hash browns
1 onion, chopped
6 eggs
1/4 cup of milk
1/2 cup of cheddar cheese, shredded
1b of ham, cubed

DIRECTIONS (PREP + COOK TIME: 35 MINUTES)

Press the sauté function and let the Ninja Foodi preheat for some minutes. Add the olive oil followed by onions and sauté them until they tenderizes. Add the hash browns and close the crisping lid. Set the Foodi to Air Crisp mode and cook for quarter-hour. Remember to open your hash brown half way. Combine the eggs with milk together in a bowl and whisk. Pour the mixture over the hash browns and cook for ten minutes. Add the cubed ham and cheese on top and allow it to rest for a minute. Serve your casserole warm.

Blueberries Breakfast Mix
INGREDIENTS (6 Servings)

2 glasses of oats
1/3 cup of brown sugar
1 teaspoon of baking powder
A teaspoon of cinnamon powder
2 cups of almond milk
2 cups of blueberries
2 tablespoons of butter
Cooking spray

DIRECTIONS (PREP + COOK TIME: 25 MINUTES)
Pour all the ingredients into a bowl and stir. Insert the reversible rack in the Foodi and place the baking pan on it. Grease it lightly with the cooking spray and add oats and blueberries. Select the bake function, set the temperature to 325°F, and cook time to 20 minutes. Transfer your blueberries mix to a bowl and ladle into serving plates. Enjoy.

Kale - Egg Frittata
INGREDIENTS (6 Servings)

11/2 cups of kale, chopped
1/4 cup of cheese, grated
6 large eggs Cooking spray
1 cup of water
2 tablespoons of heavy cream
1/2 teaspoon of nutmeg, freshly grated
Salt and pepper

DIRECTIONS (PREP + COOK TIME: 20 MINUTES)
Mix the eggs with cream, nutmeg, salt, and pepper in a bowl. Add the kale and cheese and stir to combine. Grease the cake pan lightly with cooking spray and cover the pan using an aluminum foil. Put the egg mixture in the pan. Pour some water into the pot and fix the reversible rack. Place the pan on the rack and close the lid. Press the pressure button, set the temperature to high mode, and cook time to 10 minutes. Press the start button and quick release the pressure once the set duration elapses. Subdivide your egg-frittata among six plates and enjoy.

Breakfast Quinoa
INGREDIENTS (4-6 Servings)

1 1/2 cups of quinoa, well-rinsed and drained
2 1/4 cups of broth
1 tablespoon of canola oil
2 tablespoons of maple syrup
2 teaspoons of cumin
2 teaspoons of turmeric
1/2 teaspoon of vanilla
1/4 teaspoon of ground cinnamon
Optional garnishing: chopped pecans, sliced almonds, or fresh berries

DIRECTIONS (PREP + COOK TIME: 6 MINUTES)
Add water and quinoa into the Ninja multi-cooker. Stir and add the remaining ingredients.   Close the pressure lid and set the release valve to "seal". Set the cooking time to one minute at high mode. Do a 10 minute natural-pressure release and then quick release the remaining steam. Open the lid carefully and fluff the quinoa. Serve drizzled with maple and garnish with any of the toppings.

Onion Tofu Scramble

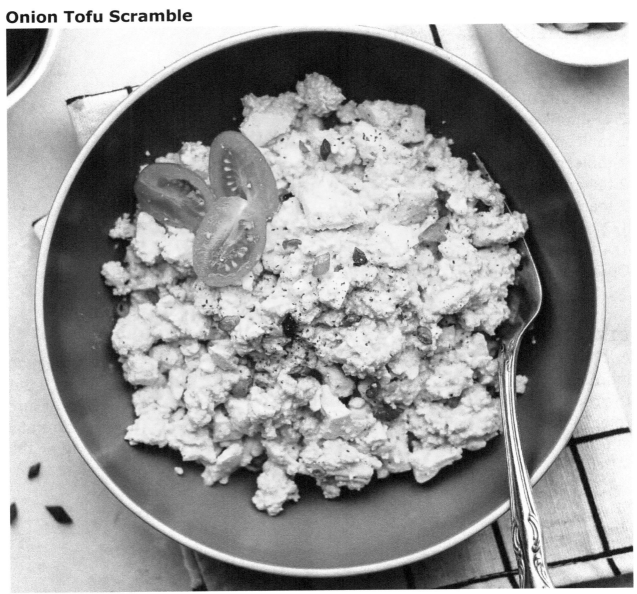

INGREDIENTS (2 Servings)

2 blocks of tofu, cubed
4 tablespoons of butter
Black pepper and salt
1 cup of cheddar cheese, grated
2 medium-sized onions, sliced

DIRECTIONS (PREP + COOK TIME: 13 MINUTES)

Combine the black pepper, salt, and tofu in a bowl. Sauté butter and onions for 3 minutes and then add the seasoned tofu. Let it cook for two minutes and add the grated cheddar cheese. Close the crisping lid and set the Foodi to air crisp mode. Set the cooking duration to 3 minutes and temperature to 340F. Serve your scramble while hot.

Scrambled Eggs
INGREDIENTS (2 Servings)

¼ cup of milk
4 whole eggs, beaten
1 tablespoon of butter
Pepper and salt

DIRECTIONS (PREP + COOK TIME: 8 MINUTES)
Whisk the eggs in the bowl and add milk. Stir the mixture until it froths. Add salt and pepper and stir again. Preheat the Foodi on Sauté and melt the butter. Add the frothed eggs and stir. Cook for 3 minutes.

Breakfast Casserole
INGREDIENTS (6 Servings)

3 cups of hash browns
1/2 lb of ground turkey-breakfast sausage
6 eggs 1/2 cup of milk
1/4 teaspoon of black pepper
1/2 teaspoon of kosher salt
1 cup of shredded Colby cheese

DIRECTIONS (PREP + COOK TIME: 30 MINUTES)
Brown the sausages on sauté mode and transfer them to a bowl. Add a cup of water to the Ninja pot and insert the reversible rack. Combine the eggs with milk, salt and pepper in the bowl. Grease the baking dish lightly and add the hash browns. Put the browned sausages into the dish and pour the egg mix over it. Sprinkle the shredded cheese over the mixture and cover it with the aluminum foil. Place the baking dish on the rack and close the crisping lid. Choose the bake/roast function and set the temperature to 375°F. Set the cooking time to 15 minutes and remember to check its progress frequently.

Bacon Veggies Combo
INGREDIENTS (4 Servings)

4 bacon slices
1 green bell pepper, seeded and chopped
1/2 cup of Monterey jack cheese
1 tablespoon of mayonnaise, preferably avocado Sautéed corn
2 scallions, chopped

DIRECTIONS (PREP + COOK TIME: 35 MINUTES)
Place the bacon slices into the basket and put it in the pot. Add the mayonnaise on top and add corn, sweet peppers, scallions, and cheese. Close the crisping lid and select the bake/roast function. Cook with a temperature of 365F for 25 minutes. Serve your combo hot.

Polenta Breakfast
INGREDIENTS (6 Servings)

1 1/2 glasses of polenta flour
1 teaspoon of salt
5 glasses of vegetable broth

DIRECTIONS (PREP + COOK TIME: 15 MINUTES)

Boil broth and salt on sear/ sauté mode. Add the polenta flour and stir. Close the pressure lid and cook o high mode for 8 minutes. Quick release the accumulated steam and open the Foodi's lid. Whisk the polenta mixture to smoothen and transfer the meal into serving plates.

Crust-less Quiche
INGREDIENTS (2 Servings)

1/2 cup of Kalamata olives, chopped
4 eggs 1/4 cup of onions, chopped
1/2 cup of milk
1/2 cup of tomatoes, chopped
1 cup of crumbled feta cheese
1 tablespoon of basil, chopped
1 tablespoon of oregano, chopped
2 tablespoons of extra-virgin olive oil
Salt and pepper

DIRECTIONS (PREP + COOK TIME: 40 MINUTES)

Smear the multi-cooker pot with organic olive oil. Beat the eggs into a bowl and add milk. Stir well and season with pepper and salt. Add the remaining ingredients and mix thoroughly. Pour the mixture into the oiled pot and close the crisping lid. Select the Air Crisp button and cook for 30 minutes at 325°F. Cool and serve.

Coconut Scramble

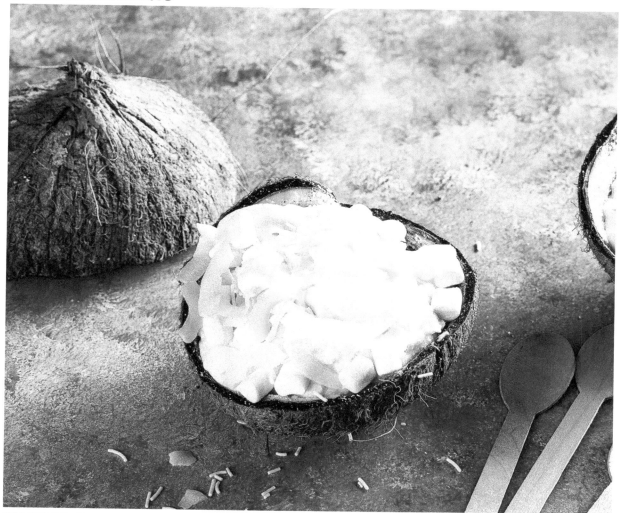

INGREDIENTS (4 Servings)

4 eggs 4 tablespoons of coconut milk
1 red onion, chopped finely
1 tablespoon of canola or coconut oil
4 tablespoons of chives
4 tablespoons of grated cheddar cheese

DIRECTIONS (PREP + COOK TIME: 25 MINUTES)

Press the sauté button on the Foodi multi-cooker. Add the oil and heat it. Add the chopped onions and stir. Sauté the contents for 3 minutes. Combine the remaining ingredients in a bowl and stir. Pour the mixture into the browned onion and toss. Press the air crisp button and cook for 10 minutes (stir after 5 minutes of cooking.) Serve the scramble while hot.

Almond and Berries Cut Oats
INGREDIENTS (4 Servings)

1 cup of cut oats
1 ½ cups of almond milk
½ cup of water
3 tablespoons of maple syrup
1 cup of mixed berries
¼ cup almonds, sliced
1 teaspoon of vanilla flavoring

DIRECTIONS (PREP + COOK TIME: 10 MINUTES)

Combine all the ingredients and close the pressure lid. Cook them for 5 minutes. Release pressure naturally for ten minutes and quick release the remaining steam. Serve the oat breakfast while hot.

Sourdough Bread
INGREDIENTS (1 Servings)

1 ½ cups of water, divided
1 ½ teaspoons of dry yeast
1 teaspoon of sugar
1 cup of plain Greek yogurt
3 cups of all-purpose flour
2 teaspoons of kosher salt
Cooking spray

DIRECTIONS (PREP + COOK TIME: 55 MINUTES)

Add yeast and sugar to a half cup of hot water and stir. Stir the sugary water for 5 minutes or until it becomes foamy. Add flour, yoghurt, and salt to the foamy mixture and mix for 2 minutes using a high-speed mixer. Preheat the multi-cooker for a minute and set it to bake/ roast mode at 250F. Shape the dough into a ball and leave it covered (in the pot) for two hours or until it rises. Place a parchment paper on the reversible rack and grease it with the cooking spray. Transfer the risen dough to the greased paper and shape it into a ball. Cover it with a towel and set aside for 15 minutes. Subdivide the dough into 4" pieces of ½" depth approximately. Pour the remaining water into the pot and insert the rack (containing the risen dough) in the Foodi. Close the crisping lid and set the multi-cooker to roast mode. Set the temperatures to 325° F and cook time to 40 minutes. After the bread is cooked, remove it from the rack and let it rest for two hours before serving.

Cheesy Meat Oatmeal
INGREDIENTS (2 Servings)

1 beef sausage, chopped
3 oz. of salami, chopped
4 slices of chopped prosciutto
1 tablespoon of ketchup
1 cup of mozzarella cheese, grated
4 eggs
1 tablespoon of chopped onion

DIRECTIONS (PREP + COOK TIME: 22 MINUTES)

Preheat your Ninja Foodi on 300°F. Set it to Air Crisp mode. Whisk the egg in a bowl. Add the ketchup and whisk. Add the onion and stir again. Grease the Foodi basket with the cooking spray. Add the sausage and cook them for two minutes or until they turn brown. Meanwhile, mix the egg mixture with the chopped salami, mozzarella cheese, and prosciutto. Pour the mixture over the sausage and stir. Close the crisping lid and let it cook for 10 minutes. Serve your meat oatmeal hot.

Breakfast Burritos
INGREDIENTS (4 Servings)

½ cup of milk
8 large eggs
¼ teaspoon of black pepper
½ teaspoon of kosher salt
1 tablespoon of extra virgin olive oil
5 oz. of fresh Mexican chorizo
1 cup of yellow onion, chopped
1 cup of poblano Chile, chopped
½ cup of water
4 ounces (about 1 cup) of Mexican cheese, blend
4 large flour tortillas
½ cup of Pico de Gallo
½ cup of fresh cilantro leaves, loosely packed

DIRECTIONS (PREP + COOK TIME: 40 MINUTES)

Mix the eggs with milk in a bowl. Add salt and pepper. Stir. Preheat the Foodi on sauté mode and cook the chorizo in oil for 5 minutes or until they brown. Add onions and poblano. Cook while stirring frequently for 5 minutes or until they tenders. Stop the sauté mode. Place the chorizo mixture on a foil-lined pan. Pour water into the Ninja Foodi and put the pan in the reversible rack. Spread the egg mixture over the chorizo mixture. Sprinkle the contents with cheese evenly. Insert the rack in the Foodi and close the pressure lid. Cook the mixture on high mode for 20 minutes. Quick release the pressure and open the pressure lid. Place tortillas on a flat surface and subdivide the egg/sausage mixture among them. Top up with two teaspoons of Pico de Gallo and two teaspoons of cilantro. Fold the tortillas' sides and roll up. Enjoy.

Maple Giant Pancake
INGREDIENTS (6 Servings)

3 cups of flour
1/2 cup of essential olive oil
1/3 cup of water
5 eggs
3/4 cup of sugar
2 tablespoon of maple syrup
1 and ½ teaspoon of baking soda
½ teaspoon of salt
A dollop of whipped cream

DIREcTIONS (PREP + COOK TIME: 35 MINUTES)

Mix the flour, eggs, sugar, water, baking soda, and salt in a bowl. Use the mixer to blend it. Pour the mixture into the Ninja Foodi and let it rest for 15 minutes. Close the lid and seal the pressure release valve. Press the pressure cook button and cook on low mode for 10 minutes. Quick release the pressure and open the lid carefully. Remove the pancake using a spatula and place it on a platter. Spread your giant pancake with maple syrup. Serve it with whipped cream toppings.

Air Fried Breakfast Sausage

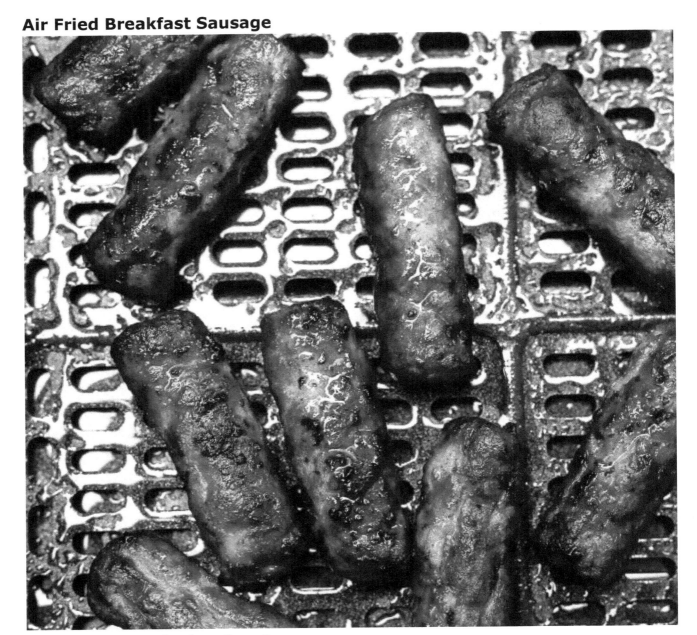

INGREDIENTS (4 Servings)

4 medium sausages
1 teaspoon of celery salt
1 teaspoon of garlic powder
 1 egg

DIRECTIONS (PREP + COOK TIME: 15 MINUTES)

Chop the sausages into mince. Add egg, celery salt, and garlic powder to the minced sausages. Form 4 patties and put them in the air crisp basket. Close the crisping lid and press the press crisp function. Set the temperature to 350°F and timer for ten minutes. Select the start/ stop button. Remove the breakfast sausage and serve.

Corned Beef Hash
INGREDIENTS (6 Servings)

1/2 lb of cooked corned beef, diced
2 tablespoons of canola oil
1 red bell pepper, chopped
1 onion (peeled and chopped)
2 medium white potatoes (peeled and diced)
3 teaspoons of salt, divided
1/2 teaspoon of ground black pepper
6 eggs

DIRECTIONS (PREP + COOK TIME: 50 MINUTES)
Sauté the corned beef. Add oil, onion, and potatoes to it. Add 2 teaspoons of salt and pepper. Sauté the seasonings until the onions brown. Cook for 5 minutes or until a crust forms at the bottom while stirring frequently. Cook for five more minutes and stir. Crack the eggs over the potatoes and close the crisping lid. Broil for 10 minutes. Serve the beef hash with hot sauce. You can also garnish with parsley.

Gold Potatoes and Bacon
INGREDIENTS (8 Servings)

2 gold potatoes, cubed
8 oz. of bacon, chopped
4 eggs, beaten
1 red bell pepper, chopped
1 yellow onion, chopped
Salt and black pepper
1 teaspoon of sweet paprika

DIRECTIONS (PREP + COOK TIME: 50 MINUTES)
Set the Foodi to sauté mode. Add the bacon and cook for 5 minutes. Add the bell pepper, onions, and gold potatoes. Sauté the mixture for 5 more minutes. Add eggs, paprika, salt, and black pepper. Set the Foodi to air fry mode and close the crisping lid. Cook the contents for thirty minutes at a temperature of 300°F. Remember to flip at around 15 minutes. Serve hot.

Simple Corned Beef Hash
INGREDIENTS (6 Servings)

2 medium cans of corned beef, diced
12 white potatoes, medium- sized
4 large carrots
1 large white onion
1and ½ cups of beef stock
1 teaspoon of parsley
Salt and pepper

DIRECTIONS (PREP + COOK TIME: 13 MINUTES)

Dice the corn beef and set aside. Prepare the vegetables by dicing the carrots, potatoes, and onions. Put the diced veggies in the Foodi and add the beef stock. Close the pressure lid on and seal the pressure valve. Cook at high mode for ten minutes. Quick release the pressure when the cooking time elapses. Open the lid and add salt and pepper. Add the diced beef and set the multi-cooker to Sauté mode. Let it cook for two minutes and serve hot.

Tuna Bowls
INGREDIENTS (4 Servings)

16 oz. of canned tuna (drained and flaked)
1 red onion, chopped
½ cup of baby spinach
2 spring onions, chopped
1 tablespoons of lime juice
3 tablespoons of melted butter

DIRECTIONS (PREP + COOK TIME: 13 MINUTES)

Set your Ninja Foodi to sauté mode and preheat it for a minute. Add butter and melt. Add onions to the butter and cook for 2 minutes while stirring. Add the remaining ingredients and stir. Close the pressure lid and set the release valve to seal position. Cook the ingredients for 5 minutes and quick release the accumulated pressure after the cooking time elapses. Subdivide the tuna bowls amongst four plates and enjoy.

Oatmeal with Carrot
INGREDIENTS (6 Servings)

1 tablespoon of butter
1 cup of cut oats
1 cup of carrots, grated
4 cups of water
1 teaspoon of pumpkin pie spice
3 tablespoons of maple syrup
¼ teaspoon of salt
¼ cup of dried apricots, chopped
½ cup of slivered almonds
½ cup of raisins

DIRECTIONS (PREP + COOK TIME: 23 MINUTES)

Put butter into the Foodi and melt it on sauté mode. Add the oats and sauté for 3 minutes while stirring consistently. Add the water, carrots, maple syrup, spices, and salt. Close the pressure lid and set the release valve to "seal." Cook the ingredients on high mode for ten minutes. Let the steam exit naturally for 10 minutes and quick release the rest. Open the pressure lid and add cinnamon, almonds, apricots, and raisins. Stir. Let your oatmeal rest for 5 minutes before serving.

Spicy Tomato Eggs

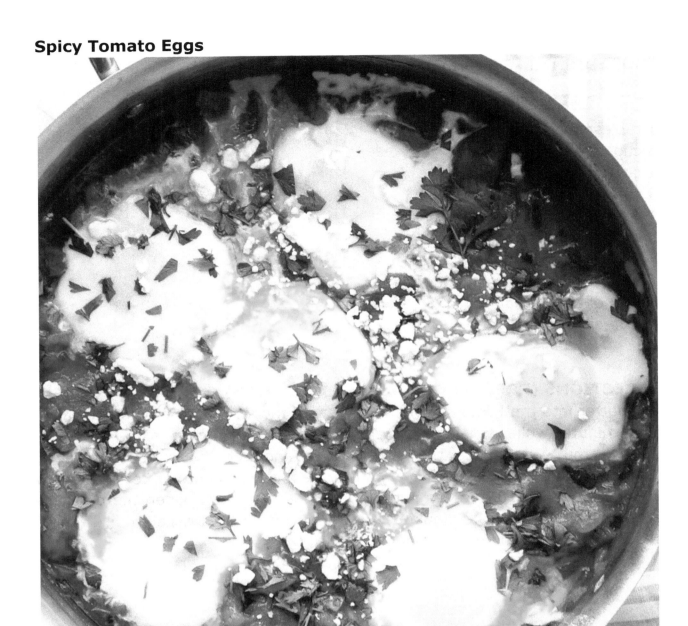

INGREDIENTS (4 Servings)

1 red bell pepper, chopped

2 tomatoes, cubed

4 eggs, whisked

1 yellow onion

2 tablespoons of organic olive oil

1 teaspoon of sweet paprika

1 teaspoon of garlic powder

1 teaspoon of onion powder
Salt and pepper

DIRECTIONS (PREP + COOK TIME: 30 MINUTES)

Set your Foodi to sauté mode and heat some olive oil. Add the bell pepper to the heated oil let it cook for five minutes while stirring occasionally. Add the cubed tomatoes, onion powder, garlic powder, paprika, salt, and pepper. Stir. Cook the ingredients for five more minutes. Add the eggs and toss well. Close the pressure lid and cook on high mode for 12 minutes. Natural-release the accumulated pressure for ten minutes. Subdivide your spiced tomato eggs amongst four plates.

Brown Rice Breakfast Risotto
INGREDIENTS (4 Servings)

2 tablespoons of butter
1 ½ cups of short grain brown rice
2 medium bananas, mashed lightly
1/3 cup of brown sugar
1 ½ teaspoons of cinnamon
½ teaspoon of salt
3 cups of light coconut milk
1 cup of dry white wine
Chopped walnuts

DIRECTIONS (PREP + COOK TIME: 30 MINUTES)

Smear some butter on your Foodi's base and melt it on sauté mode. Add the rice and cook for two minutes while stirring constantly. Add the bananas, cinnamon, salt, sugar, milk, and wine. Close the pressure lid and cook on high mode for 22 minutes. Natural-release the in-built pressure and serve with chopped walnuts garnishing.

Turkey Burrito
INGREDIENTS (2 Servings)

1 turkey breast (cooked and shredded)
3 eggs, whisked
1 red pepper, sliced
1 avocado (peeled, pitted, and sliced)
Salt and pepper
2 tablespoons of shredded mozzarella cheese
2 corn tortillas
Cooking spray

DIRECTIONS (PREP + COOK TIME: 11 MINUTES)

Smear the pan with the cooking spray. Add salt, pepper, and the whisked eggs into a pan and mix. Add the remaining ingredients except cheese and tortilla. Whisk well. Fix the reversible rack in the pot and place a pan on it. Cover the pan's content with a foil and closes the pressure lid. Cook on high mode for10 minutes and then quick release the accumulated steam. Place the tortillas on a clean surface and subdivide the egg mixture equally amongst them. Top each of them with mozzarella cheese and enjoy

Cauliflower Mix
INGREDIENTS (4 Servings)

1 ½ cups of white cauliflower, florets separated
1 ½ cups of purple cauliflower, florets separated
 2 garlic cloves, minced.
½ cup of peas
1 carrot, cubed.
2 spring onions, chopped
2 and ½ teaspoons of soy sauce
2 teaspoons of organic olive oil
A pinch of salt and black pepper

DIRECTIONS (PREP + COOK TIME: 20 MINUTES)

Set the Foodi to Sauté mode and add oil. Heat it up. Add the onions and garlic and stir. Cook for three minutes.   Add the carrots, cauliflower, soy sauce, salt, pepper, and peas. Toss and close the pressure lid. Cook on high mode for 8 minutes. Release the pressure naturally for ten minutes. Subdivide your cauliflower mix between plates as a side dish.

Potato Salad
INGREDIENTS (6 Servings)

2 lb of red potatoes, scrubbed
1 yellow onion, chopped
5 bacon strips, chopped
2 celery stalks, chopped
¼ cup of apple cider vinegar
1 cup of sauerkraut
½ cup of scallions, chopped
½ cup of water
1 tablespoon of mustard
¼ teaspoon of sweet paprika
1 teaspoon of sugar
A pinch of salt and black pepper

DIRECTIONS (PREP + COOK TIME: 25 MINUTES)
Put the potatoes and water into the Ninja Foodi and close the pressure lid. Cook on high mode for 5 minutes and release the pressure naturally for 10 minutes Cool the potatoes, peel, and cube them. Clean the Foodi and set it to sauté mode. Add the bacon and stir. Cook for 5 minutes Add the onions and stir. Cook for another 5 minutes. Add vinegar and toss. Cook for one minute. Add the scrubbed potatoes and the remaining ingredients. Toss and cook until the potatoes soften. Subdivide your potato salad between plates as a side dish.

Garlicky Broccoli
INGREDIENTS (4 Servings)

1 broccoli head, florets separated
3 garlic cloves, minced
2 tablespoons of lemon juice
2 tablespoons of parsley, chopped
1 tablespoon of essential olive oil

DIRECTIONS (PREP + COOK TIME: 30 MINUTES)
Set the Foodi on sauté mode and add oil. Heat it up. Add the garlic, broccoli, and lemon juice. Toss and cook for two minutes   Close the pressure lid and cook on high mode for 15 minutes. Let the accumulated pressure release for 10 minutes naturally. Subdivide your garlicky broccoli between serving plates as a side dish.

Easy Gnocchi

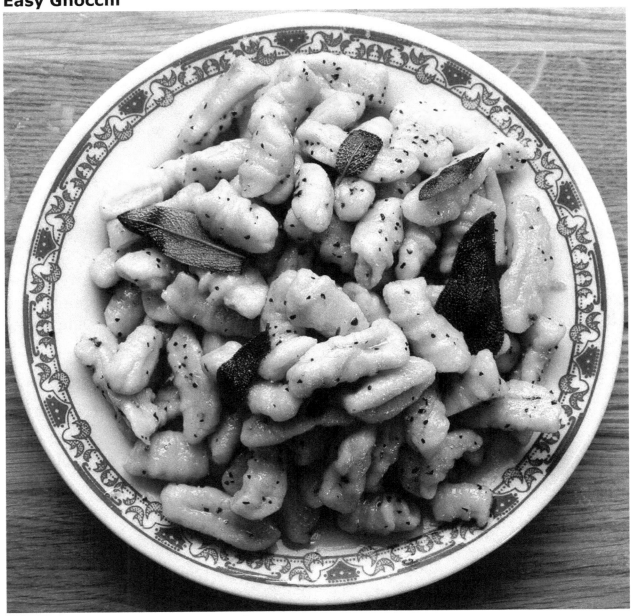

INGREDIENTS (6 Servings)

50 oz. of potato gnocchi
10 oz. of baby spinach
½ cup of goat cheese, crumbled
¼ cup of parmesan, grated
1/3 cup of white flour
3 and ½ cups of heavy cream

1 ½ cups of chicken stock
A pinch of salt and black pepper

DIRECTIONS (PREP + COOK TIME: 32 MINUTES)

Set the Foodi to Sauté mode and heat it up. Add the stock, cream, flour, salt, pepper, and nutmeg. Whisk well and cook for 8 minutes.   Add the spinach and gnocchi. Sprinkle the mixture with parmesan and goat cheese. Set the Foodi to bake mode and cook at 325 °F for 15 minutes. Subdivide your gnocchi side dish amongst plates.

Warm Potato Salad
INGREDIENTS (4 Servings)

2 gold potatoes cut into wedges
3 tablespoons of heavy cream
1 tablespoon of canola oil
Salt and black pepper

DIRECTIONS (PREP + COOK TIME: 30 MINUTES)

Put the potatoes in the air crisp basket and insert it in the Foodi. Set the multi-cooker to air crisp mode and cook at 400 °F for 10 minutes   Transfer the potatoes to a bowl and clean the Foodi. Set it to sauté mode and add oil. Heat it up. Put the potato wedges, salt, pepper, and cream into the pot. Toss and cook for 10 minutes. Subdivide your salad between plates as a side dish

Zucchini Fries
INGREDIENTS (4 Servings)

2 small zucchinis cut into fries
2 eggs, whisked
1 cup of bread crumbs
½ cup of white flour
Cooking spray
Salt and black pepper

DIRECTIONS (PREP + COOK TIME: 22 MINUTES)

Mix flour, salt, and pepper in a bowl. Stir. Put the breadcrumbs in another bowl and add the whisked eggs. Dredge the zucchini fries in the bread crumb mixture and transfer them to the Foodi's air crisp basket. Fix the basket in the Foodi and grease the fries with the cooking spray. Set the multi-cooker to air crisp mode and cook at 400 °F for 12 minutes. Subdivide your zucchini side dish between plates.

Veggie Side Salad
INGREDIENTS (4 Servings)

1 eggplant, cubed
1 green bell pepper, chopped
1 bunch of cilantro, chopped
2 garlic cloves, minced
1 yellow onion, chopped
1 tablespoon of tomato sauce
1 tablespoon of extra virgin olive oil
Salt and black pepper

DIRECTIONS (PREP + COOK TIME: 22 MINUTES)

Set the Foodi to Sauté mode and add the oil. Heat it up. Add all the ingredients (except the cilantro) and toss. Close the pressure lid and cook on high mode for 12 minutes. Release pressure naturally for 10 minutes. Subdivide your veggie side dish between plates and enjoy.

Sumac Eggplant
INGREDIENTS (6 Servings)

2 lb of eggplants, cubed
1 tablespoon of organic olive oil
1 teaspoon of sumac
1 teaspoon of garlic powder
Juice extracted from a lime.

DIRECTIONS (PREP + COOK TIME: 25 MINUTES)
Set the Foodi to sauté mode and add oil. Heat it up. Add the eggplant, garlic powder, sumac, and lime juice. Toss and close the pressure lid. Cook on high mode for 15 minutes. Release the pressure for 10 minutes naturally. Subdivide the eggplant mixture between plates as a side dish.

Thyme Red Potatoes
INGREDIENTS (4 Servings)

4 red potatoes, thinly sliced
1 tablespoon of organic olive oil
2 teaspoons of thyme, chopped
Salt and black pepper

DIRECTIONS (PREP + COOK TIME: 40 MINUTES)
Mix all the ingredients in a bowl and toss. Transfer the mixture to an air crisp basket and insert it in the Foodi. Set the multi-cooker to air crisp mode and cook at 370 °F for 30 minutes. Subdivide your thyme-potatoes between serving plates as a side dish

Cauliflower and Pineapple Salad

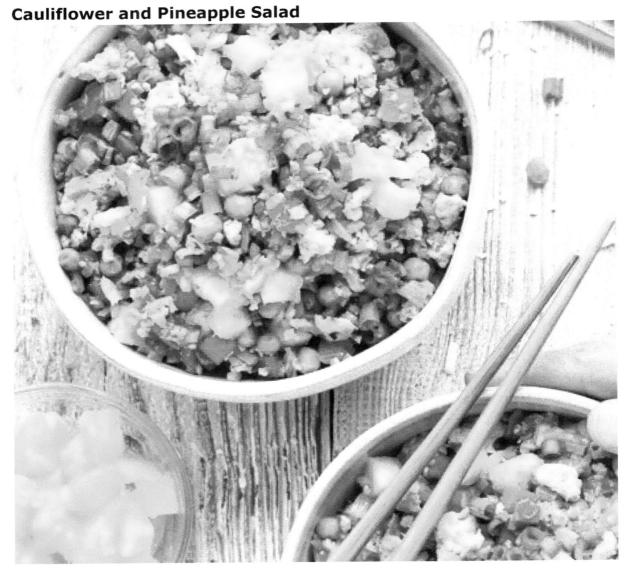

INGREDIENTS (6 Servings)

2 cauliflower florets

1 pineapple (peeled and cubed)

1 mango (peeled and cubed)

1 cup of chicken stock, heated up

2 teaspoons of essential olive oil

Salt and black pepper

DIRECTIONS (PREP + COOK TIME: 30 MINUTES) Set the Foodi to sauté mode and add the oil. Heat it up and add the cauliflower. Cook for 5 minutes. Add the remaining ingredients to the pot and close the pressure lid. Cook on high mode for 15 minutes and release the steam naturally for 10 minutes. Subdivide your pineapple salad between serving plates as a side dish.

Hazelnut Cauliflower Rice
INGREDIENTS (4 Servings)

1 spring onion, chopped
2 garlic cloves, minced
2 cups of cauliflower rice
2 cups of chicken stock
½ cup of hazelnuts (toasted and chopped)
1 tablespoon of cilantro (chopped)
1 teaspoon of essential olive oil
Salt and black pepper

DIRECTIONS (PREP + COOK TIME: 32 MINUTES)
Set the Foodi to Sauté mode and add the oil. Warm it and add onions. Add the minced garlic and stir. Cook for 3 minutes. Add the cauliflower rice, stock, hazelnuts, salt, and pepper. Toss and close the pressure lid. Cook on high mode for 20 minutes. Release the accumulated steam naturally for 10 minutes. Add the chopped cilantro and toss. Subdivide your cauliflower rice between serving plates as a side dish.

Maple Carrots
INGREDIENTS (6 Servings)

2 lbs of carrots, roughly cubed
1 tablespoon of canola oil
2 tablespoon of maple syrup
1 tablespoon of parsley, chopped

DIRECTIONS (PREP + COOK TIME: 25 MINUTES)
Mix all the ingredients in a bowl and transfer the mixture into an air crisp basket. Fit the basket in the Foodi and set it to crisping mode. Cook at 350 °F for 20 minutes. Subdivide the maple carrots between serving plates as a side dish.

Green Beans Salad
INGREDIENTS (4 Servings)

1 ½ lb of green beans, trimmed
½ lb of shallots, chopped
¼ cup of walnuts, chopped
2 tablespoons of olive oil
Salt and black pepper

DIRECTIONS (PREP + COOK TIME: 30 MINUTES)
Combine all the ingredients in the crisping basket and fix it in the Foodi Set the multi-cooker to air crisp mode and cook at 360 °F for 20 minutes. Subdivide your beans' salad between serving plates as a side dish.

Roasted Tomato Salad
INGREDIENTS (2 Servings)

20 oz. of cherry tomatoes, cut into quarters
½ cup of cilantro
1 white onion, roughly chopped
 1 jalapeno pepper, chopped
 Juice extracted from one lime
1 tablespoon of extra virgin olive oil
Salt and black pepper

DIRECTIONS (PREP + COOK TIME: 16 MINUTES)
Set the Foodi to sauté mode and add the oil. Heat it and add the onions. Stir and sauté the onions for three minutes.   Add the remaining ingredients and toss. Set the Ninja Foodi to roast mode and cook at 380 °F for 4 minutes. Subdivide your tomato salad between serving plates as a side dish.

Potato Mash
INGREDIENTS (4 Servings)

3 gold potatoes (peeled and cubed)
½ cup of cheddar cheese, shredded
1 cup of heavy cream
1 cup of water
¼ cup of butter, melted
A pinch of salt and black pepper

DIRECTIONS (PREP + COOK TIME: 20 MINUTES)
Put the potatoes and water in the Foodi and close the pressure lid. Cook on high mode for ten minutes and release the pressure naturally for another ten minutes. Drain the potatoes and transfer them to a bowl. Mash them and add butter, cheese, cream, salt, and pepper. Stir. Subdivide your potato mash between serving plates as a side dish.

Spiced Squash

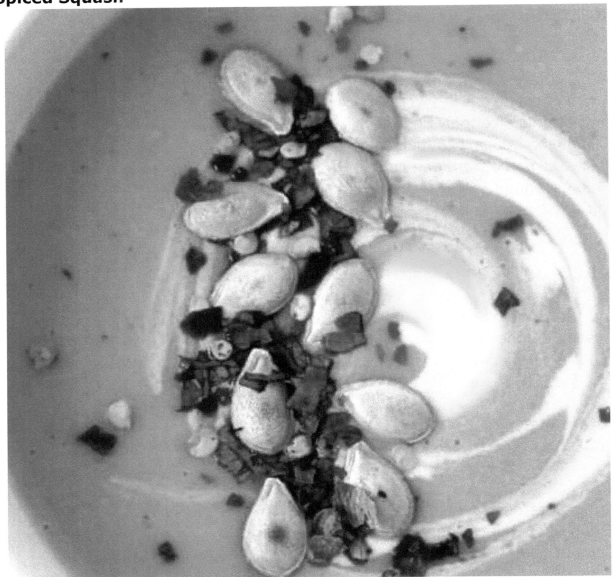

INGREDIENTS (4 Servings)

6 oz of squash, cubed
2 oz of heavy cream
1 small yellow onion, chopped
2 garlic cloves, minced
2 tablespoons of extra virgin olive oil
½ teaspoon of cinnamon powder
½ teaspoon of allspice

½ teaspoon of nutmeg, ground
½ teaspoon of ginger, grated

DIRECTIONS (PREP + COOK TIME: 25 MINUTES)

Set the Foodi to sauté mode and add the oil. Heat it up. Add onions and garlic. Stir and cook for 5 minutes. Add the remaining ingredients and toss. Set the Foodi to baking mode and cook everything at 360 °F for fifteen minutes. Subdivide your squash between serving plates as a side dish.

Beans and Tomatoes Mix
INGREDIENTS (6 Servings)

1 lb of canned red kidney beans, drained
½ lb of cherry tomatoes, cut into quarters
1 yellow onion, chopped
4 garlic cloves, chopped
2 spring onions, minced
1 teaspoon of essential olive oil
2 tablespoons of cilantro, minced
2 tablespoons of tomato sauce
Salt and black pepper

DIRECTIONS (PREP + COOK TIME: 30 MINUTES)

Mix all the ingredients (except cilantro) in your Foodi's baking pan and toss. Insert the reversible rack in the equipment and place the baking pan on it. Set the Foodi to baking mode and cook everything for 20 minutes. Add the minced cilantro and stir. Subdivide your tomatoes side dish between plates and enjoy.

Potatoes and Tomatoes
INGREDIENTS (6 Servings)

15 oz of potatoes, cubed
6 oz of canned tomatoes, chopped
2 spring onions, chopped
2 tablespoons of extra virgin olive oil
½ teaspoon of nutmeg, ground
Salt and black pepper

DIRECTIONS (PREP + COOK TIME: 25 MINUTES)

Set the Foodi to sauté mode and add the oil. Heat it up and add the onions. Stir and cook for 3 minutes. Add the potatoes, nutmeg, tomatoes, salt, and pepper to the onions. Toss and close the pressure lid. Cook on high mode for fifteen minutes. Release the accumulated vapor naturally for ten minutes. Subdivide the side dish between plates and enjoy.

Creamy Cauliflower
INGREDIENTS (4 Servings)

1 cauliflower head, florets separated
½ cup of Italian bread crumbs
¼ cup of raisins
½ cup of heavy cream
½ cup of parmesan, grated
1 cup of beer
1 tablespoon of white flour
A teaspoon of nutmeg, ground
A pinch of salt and black pepper

DIRECTIONS (PREP + COOK TIME: 25 MINUTES)
Combine beer with the raisins, cauliflower, salt, pepper, and nutmeg in your Foodi. Toss and close the pressure lid. Cook the ingredients on high mode for 3 minutes. Release the pressure naturally for four minutes and quick release the rest. Add the cream mixed with the flour and toss. Set the Foodi to sauté mode and continue cooking for 5 more minutes. Mix the bread crumbs with cheese in a bowl. Stir and pour it over the cauliflower mixture. Close the crisping lid and set the Foodi to air crisp mode. Cook at 390 °F for ten minutes. Subdivide your creamy cauliflower between serving plates as a side dish.

Garlic Mushrooms
INGREDIENTS (4 Servings)

1 lb of brown mushrooms, halved
1 tablespoon of garlic, minced
A tablespoon of lime juice
1 tablespoon of chives, chopped
2 tablespoons of extra virgin olive oil
Salt and black pepper

DIRECTIONS (PREP + COOK TIME: 30 MINUTES)

Set the Foodi to sauté mode and add the oil. Warm it and add garlic and mushrooms. Toss and sauté for 5 minutes. Add the lime juice and set the multi-cooker to baking mode. Cook at 380 °F for 15 minutes. Add the chives and toss. Subdivide the mushroom side dish between serving plates and enjoy.

Sweet Potato and Mayo
INGREDIENTS (2 Servings)

2 sweet potatoes (peeled and cut into wedges)
4 tablespoons of mayonnaise
2 tablespoons of organic olive oil
½ teaspoon of curry powder
¼ teaspoon of coriander, ground
½ teaspoon of cumin, ground
A pinch of ginger powder
Salt and black pepper

DIRECTIONS (PREP + COOK TIME: 30 MINUTES)

Mix the sweet potato wedges with salt, pepper, coriander, curry powder, and oil in the crisping basket. Toss well. Insert the basket in the Foodi and set it to air crisp mode. Cook the potatoes at 380 °F for 20 minutes. Remember to shake the pot at the 10th minute. Transfer the potatoes to a bowl and add the remaining ingredients. Toss and serve as a side dish.

Yummy Eggplant

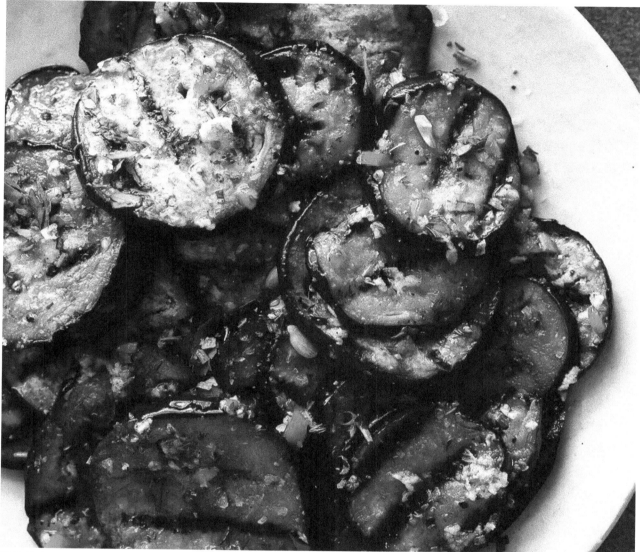

INGREDIENTS (4 Servings)

4 eggplants (cut into cubes)
1 red onion, chopped
1 tablespoon of smoked paprika
1 tablespoon of organic olive oil
Salt and black pepper

DIRECTIONS (PREP + COOK TIME: 25 MINUTES)

Set the Foodi to Sauté mode and add the oil. Heat it up and add the eggplants followed by the remaining ingredients. Stir. Close the pressure lid and cook on high mode for fifteen minutes. Release the pressure naturally for 10 minutes. Subdivide your yummy eggplants between serving plates as a side dish.

Buttery Brussels sprouts
INGREDIENTS (8 Servings)

3 lbs of Brussels sprouts, trimmed
1 lb of bacon, chopped
1 yellow onion, chopped
2 cups of heavy cream
4 tablespoons of butter, melted
1 teaspoon of extra virgin olive oil
 Salt and black pepper

DIRECTIONS (PREP + COOK TIME: 30 MINUTES)
Put the Brussels sprouts in the crisping basket and insert it in your Ninja Foodi. Set it to air crisp mode and cook at 370 °F for 10 minutes. Transfer the cooked sprouts to a bowl and clean the Foodi. Set the multi-cooker to sauté mode and add oil and butter. Heat it to melt the butter. Return the sprouts to the Foodi and add the chopped bacon. Add onions and stir. Continue cooking the ingredients for five more minutes. Subdivide the sprouts between plates as a side dish.

Asian Style Chickpeas
INGREDIENTS (4 Servings)

30 oz of canned chickpeas, drained
2 tablespoons of olive oil
2 teaspoons of garam Masala
¼ teaspoon of mustard powder
½ teaspoon of garlic powder
1 teaspoon of sweet paprika
A pinch of salt and black pepper

DIRECTIONS (PREP + COOK TIME: 30 MINUTES)
Mix all the ingredients in a bowl and toss well. Set the Ninja Foodi to sauté mode and heat it up for 3 minutes. Add the chickpeas mixture and sauté them for 6 minutes Transfer them to the Foodi's basket and set it to air crisp mode. Cook the mixture at 400 °F for fifteen minutes. Subdivide your chickpeas side dish between plates as a side dish.

Brussels sprouts
INGREDIENTS (4 Servings)

1 lb of Brussels sprouts, halved
4 bacon strips (cooked and chopped)
1 tablespoon of extra virgin olive oil
2 teaspoons of garlic powder
A pinch of salt and black pepper

DIRECTIONS (PREP + COOK TIME: 25 MINUTES)
Mix all the ingredients in a bowl (except bacon) and toss. Put the Brussels sprouts in the crisping basket and set it to air crisp mode. Cook at 390 °F for twenty minutes. Subdivide the Brussels sprouts between plates and top them with bacon.

Sweet Potato Mash
INGREDIENTS (4 Servings)

1 ½ lbs of sweet potatoes (peeled and cubed)
1 cup of chicken stock
1 tablespoon of honey
A tablespoon of butter, softened
Salt and black pepper

DIRECTIONS (PREP + COOK TIME: 20 MINUTES)

Mix the sweet potatoes with stock, salt, and pepper in your Foodi. Close the pressure lid and cook for 15 minutes. Release the pressure naturally for ten minutes Mash the potatoes and add the softened butter followed by honey. Whisk well and subdivide the mash between serving plates as a side dish.

Carrot Puree
INGREDIENTS (4 Servings)

1 lb of carrots (peeled and halved) A yellow onion, chopped
½ cup of chicken stock
¼ cup of heavy cream
Salt and black pepper

DIRECTIONS (PREP + COOK TIME: 25 MINUTES)

Mix all the ingredients (except cream) in your Ninja Foodi. Close the pressure lid and cook on high mode for 15 minutes. Release the accumulated vapor naturally for ten minutes Mash everything and add cream. Whisk. Subdivide your carrot puree between plates as a side dish.

Roasted Potatoes

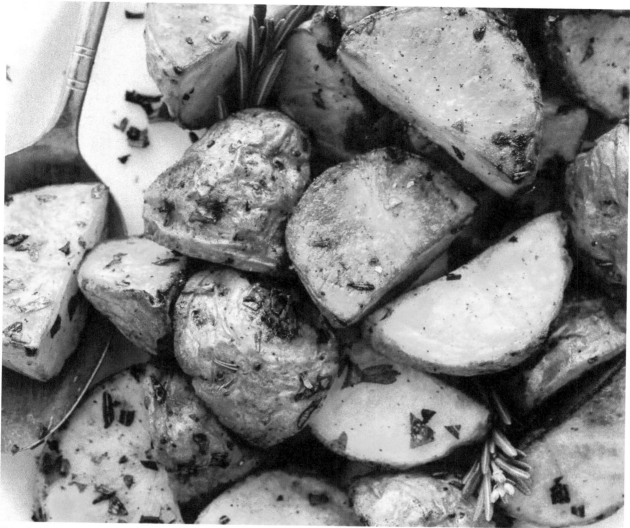

INGREDIENTS (4 Servings)

1 lb of baby potatoes, halved
½ cup of parsley, chopped
½ cup of mayonnaise
2 tablespoons of tomato paste
2 tablespoons of extra virgin olive oil
1 tablespoons of smoked paprika
A tablespoon of garlic powder
2 tablespoons of white wine vinegar
3 teaspoons of hot paprika
A pinch of salt and black pepper

DIRECTIONS (PREP + COOK TIME: 35 MINUTES)

Combine the potatoes with hot paprika, oil, smoked paprika, garlic powder, salt, and pepper in a bowl. Toss well. Put the potatoes in the crisping basket and insert it in the Foodi. Set the multi-cooker to air crisp mode and cook the potatoes at 360 °F for 25 minutes. Transfer the mixture to a bowl and add tomato paste, mayo, vinegar, and parsley. Toss your roasted potatoes and serve as a side dish.

Cauliflower Risotto
INGREDIENTS (4 Servings)

1 cauliflower head, diced
15 oz of water chestnuts, drained
1 egg, whisked
A tablespoon of ginger, grated
1 tablespoon of freshly squeezed lemon juice
2 tablespoons of olive oil
4 tablespoons of soy sauce
3 garlic cloves, minced

DIRECTIONS (PREP + COOK TIME: 32 MINUTES)

Set the Foodi to sauté mode and add the oil. Heat it up. Add the minced garlic and cauliflower rice. Toss and cook for three minutes. Add soy sauce, chestnuts, and ginger. Toss and close the pressure lid. Cook on high mode for 15 minutes. Release the accumulated pressure naturally for four minutes and quick release the rest for a minute. Set the Ninja Foodi to sauté mode and add the egg. Stir well and cook for 2 more minutes. Subdivide your risotto between plates and serve as a side dish.

Creamy Artichokes
INGREDIENTS (4 Servings)

15 oz of canned artichoke hearts
1 ½ tablespoons of thyme, chopped
2 garlic cloves, minced
1 yellow onion, chopped
A cup of heavy cream
1 tablespoon of olive oil
1 tablespoon of parmesan, grated
Salt and black pepper

DIRECTIONS (PREP + COOK TIME: 30 MINUTES)

Set the Foodi to sauté mode and add the oil. Heat it. Add onions and garlic. Stir the seasonings and sauté for 5 minutes. Add the remaining ingredients (except the thyme and parmesan) and toss. Set the Foodi to baking mode and cook at 370 °F for 15 minutes. Spread parmesan and thyme and continue baking for five more minutes. Subdivide your creamy artichoke between plates and serve.

Conclusion

Did you take pleasure in trying these brand-new as well as delicious dishes? However we have come to the end of this cookbook regarding the use of the superb Ninja Foodi multi-cooker, which I really hope you appreciated.

To boost your health and wellness we want to advise you to incorporate physical activity and a dynamic way of living along with complying with these fantastic recipes, so regarding emphasize the renovations. we will certainly be back soon with an increasing number of appealing vegan recipes, a big hug, see you soon.

9 781008 951518